Table of Contents

Introduction

Fasting is the willful refrainment from eating and drinking. In a physiological context, fasting may refer to the metabolic status of a person who has not eaten overnight, or to the metabolic state achieved after complete digestion and absorption of a meal. Several metabolic adjustments occur during fasting. Some diagnostic tests are used to determine a fasting state. For example, a person is assumed to be fasting once 8–12 hours have elapsed since the last meal. Metabolic changes of the fasting state begin after absorption of a meal (typically 3–5 hours after eating).

A diagnostic fast refers to prolonged fasting from 1 to 100 hours (depending on age) conducted under observation to facilitate the investigation of a health complication, usually hypoglycemia. Many people may also fast as part of a medical procedure or a check-up, such as preceding a colonoscopy or surgery.

Fasting is the willful refrainment from eating and drinking. In a physiological context, fasting may refer to the metabolic status of a person who has not eaten overnight, or to the metabolic state achieved after complete digestion and absorption of a meal. Several metabolic adjustments occur during fasting. Some diagnostic tests are used to determine a fasting state. For example, a person is assumed to be fasting once 8–12 hours have elapsed since the last meal. Metabolic changes of the fasting state begin after absorption of a meal (typically 3–5 hours after eating).

A diagnostic fast refers to prolonged fasting from 1 to 100 hours (depending on age) conducted under observation to facilitate the investigation of a health complication, usually hypoglycemia. Many people may also fast as part of a medical procedure or a check-up, such as preceding a colonoscopy or surgery.

Is intermittent fasting safe for diabetes?

Intermittent fasting may present some risks for people with diabetes.

If you use insulin or medications and suddenly eat much less than normal, blood sugar can drop too low. This is called hypoglycemia.

According to the American Diabetes Association (ADA), hypoglycemia can lead to symptoms such as:

- shakiness
- confusion
- irritability
- rapid heartbeat
- feeling nervous
- sweating
- chills
- dizziness
- sleepiness
- low energy
- blurred vision
- nausea

Another potential danger of intermittent fasting with diabetes is high blood sugar. This is known as hyperglycemia.

Hyperglycemia can happen if you eat more than you typically do, which may be likely to occur if you're especially hungry after a period of fasting.

High blood sugar levels can increase your risk of diabetes complications, such as:

- nerve damage (neuropathy)
- eye conditions and blindness
- kidney disease
- heart disease
- stroke
- high blood pressure

Before starting any diet or weight loss plan, consider meeting with a member of your diabetes care team, such as a physician or dietitian, to make sure it's safe for you.

Can intermittent fasting cause diabetes?

Some early research on animals shows that intermittent fasting may impact the pancreas and insulin resistance, but more studies are needed to determine its impact on diabetes in humans.

A 2020 study looked at what happened to rats when they fasted every other day for 12 weeks. It found that the rats had an increase in belly fat, damage to pancreas cells that release insulin, and signs of insulin resistance.

It's important to note that the findings may be different if humans took part in the same experiment. More research is needed to determine whether intermittent fasting can increase the risk of diabetes in people.

Can intermittent fasting reverse diabetes?

It may be possible for intermittent fasting to put diabetes into remission for some people, perhaps due to weight loss.

A 2018 case report evaluated three people with type 2 diabetes who used insulin and fasted at least three times a week. Within a month, they no longer needed to use insulin.

They also had improvements in their body mass index (BMI), waist circumference, and HbA1C levels. After several months, the participants each lost about 10 percent of their body weight.

The sample size of that report was too small to make conclusions about how intermittent fasting can affect the majority of people with diabetes.

However, a larger study in 2018 found that nearly half of people with type 2 diabetes who lost weight were able to stop using diabetes medication and achieve remission.

Since intermittent fasting can be a way to cut calories, it may help people with diabetes lose weight and increase their likelihood of remission.

Other weight loss strategies may also help reverse diabetes, however.

Everyone is different, so what's best for you may differ from what works best for someone else. Consult with a healthcare professional or dietitian to determine which strategy may be right for you.

What is intermittent fasting?

Fasting is when you stop eating or drinking (or both) for a stretch of time. People may fast for a variety of reasons, such as:

- as a religious practice
- in preparation for a medical procedure
- an attempt to lose weight
- to improve health in some way

Intermittent fasting is an eating pattern that involves periods of eating little to no food, followed by regular meals. Unlike many other diets, it usually focuses on restricting the timing of when you eat and drink, rather than the foods on your plate.

Intermittent fasting is often used as a way to lose weight through calorie restriction. It may provide certain benefits for people with diabetes, but there are risks involved.

Types of intermittent fasting diets for diabetes

While intermittent fasting diets come in a variety of styles, no particular one has been proven best for people with diabetes.

Here are a few common intermittent fasting diets:

16:8 intermittent fasting. People following this diet eat all meals within an 8-hour window, followed by 16 hours of fasting. Many people fast from 8 p.m. until noon the next day, and keep their eating window between noon and 8 p.m.

5:2 intermittent fasting. This is when you eat regular meals for 5 days, then have 2 days of fasting, during which you eat fewer than 500 calories per day.

Alternate-day fasting. This is a full 24 hours without eating anything or only eating a small amount, followed by 24 hours of eating as usual.

Early time-restricted feeding (eTRF). This restricts your mealtimes to the morning and early afternoon, followed by a fast that lasts the rest of the day and night.

What are the benefits of intermittent fasting for diabetes?

When done safely, intermittent fasting may provide some benefits for people with diabetes. If the eating plan leads to weight loss, people may be able to reduce the amount of diabetes medication they take.

Some people have been able to stop using insulin after fasting intermittently for a month or so, according to the small study on three people mentioned earlier.

More research is needed to determine if intermittent fasting can help most people with diabetes stop using insulin.

Other potential benefits include:

- improved insulin sensitivity

- lower blood pressure

- lower oxidative stress

- reduced appetite

- increased fat oxidation

More research is needed to determine the long-term benefits of intermittent fasting on glucose control and diabetes complications, according to the ADA.

Tips for intermittent fasting when you have diabetes

If you have diabetes and are thinking of trying intermittent fasting, here are some tips:

Talk with your healthcare provider about adjusting medication or insulin dosages. You may need to change your diabetes treatment when trying a diet that could affect your blood sugar levels.

Monitor your blood sugar levels. Long periods without eating can cause blood sugar to go too low, so check you glucose levels often.

Check in on your mood. Many people find that restricting food intake can really affect their mood. Watch for signs like irritability, increased anxiety, and difficulty coping with stress.

Monitor energy levels. Fasting can make you feel fatigued — something you might want to keep in mind if you're driving or operating equipment.

Balance your carbohydrates. Your body breaks down carbohydrates into glucose, which can lead to a spike in blood sugar. When you're not fasting, try to balance carbohydrates in your meals with vegetables and protein to avoid high blood sugar.

The takeaway

Intermittent fasting can be one way to lose weight, which may help you manage diabetes.

One case study showed that intermittent fasting helped a few people with diabetes stop using insulin. Still, more research is needed.

While intermittent fasting can be done safely, people with diabetes may be at risk of hypoglycemia and hyperglycemia, due to fluctuations in blood sugar during and after periods of not eating.

Work with a healthcare professional, a member of your diabetes care team, or a dietitian before starting any weight loss plan. They can help you lose weight safely and sustainably.

Health Benefits of Fasting, Backed by Science

Despite its recent surge in popularity, fasting is a practice that dates back centuries and plays a central role in many cultures and religions.

Defined as the abstinence from all or some foods or drinks for a set period of time, there are many different ways of fasting.

In general, most types of fasts are performed over 24–72 hours.

Intermittent fasting, on the other hand, involves cycling between periods of eating and fasting, ranging from a few hours to a few days at a time.

Fasting has been shown to have many health benefits, from increased weight loss to better brain function.

Here are 8 health benefits of fasting — backed by science.

1. Promotes Blood Sugar Control by Reducing Insulin Resistance

Several studies have found that fasting may improve blood sugar control, which could be especially useful for those at risk of diabetes.

In fact, one study in 10 people with type 2 diabetes showed that short-term intermittent fasting significantly decreased blood sugar levels.

Meanwhile, another review found that both intermittent fasting and alternate-day fasting were as effective as limiting calorie intake at reducing insulin resistance.

Decreasing insulin resistance can increase your body's sensitivity to insulin, allowing it to transport glucose from your bloodstream to your cells more efficiently.

Coupled with the potential blood sugar-lowering effects of fasting, this could help keep your blood sugar steady, preventing spikes and crashes in your blood sugar levels.

Keep in mind though that some studies have found that fasting may impact blood sugar levels differently for men and women.

For instance, one small, three-week study showed that practicing alternate-day fasting impaired blood sugar control in women but had no effect in men.

Summary

Intermittent fasting and alternate-day fasting could help decrease blood sugar levels and reduce insulin resistance but may affect men and women differently.

2. Promotes Better Health by Fighting Inflammation

While acute inflammation is a normal immune process used to help fight off infections, chronic inflammation can have serious consequences for your health.

Research shows that inflammation may be involved in the development of chronic conditions, such as heart disease, cancer and rheumatoid arthritis.

Some studies have found that fasting can help decrease levels of inflammation and help promote better health.

One study in 50 healthy adults showed that intermittent fasting for one month significantly decreased levels of inflammatory markers.

Another small study discovered the same effect when people fasted for 12 hours a day for one month.

What's more, one animal study found that following a very low-calorie diet to mimic the effects of fasting reduced levels of inflammation and was beneficial in the treatment of multiple sclerosis, a chronic inflammatory condition.

Summary

Some studies have found that fasting could decrease several markers of inflammation and may be useful in treating inflammatory conditions, such as multiple sclerosis.

3. May Enhance Heart Health by Improving Blood Pressure, Triglycerides and Cholesterol Levels

Heart disease is considered the leading cause of death around the world, accounting for an estimated 31.5% of deaths globally.

Switching up your diet and lifestyle is one of the most effective ways to reduce your risk of heart disease.

Some research has found that incorporating fasting into your routine may be especially beneficial when it comes to heart health.

One small study revealed that eight weeks of alternate-day fasting reduced levels of "bad" LDL cholesterol and blood triglycerides by 25% and 32% respectively.

Another study in 110 obese adults showed that fasting for three weeks under medical supervision significantly decreased blood pressure, as well as levels of blood triglycerides, total cholesterol and "bad" LDL cholesterol.

In addition, one study in 4,629 people associated fasting with a lower risk of coronary artery disease, as well as a significantly lower risk of diabetes, which is a major risk factor for heart disease.

Summary

Fasting has been associated with a lower risk of coronary heart disease and may help lower blood pressure, triglycerides and cholesterol levels.

4. May Boost Brain Function and Prevent Neurodegenerative Disorders

Though research is mostly limited to animal research, several studies have found that fasting could have a powerful effect on brain health.

One study in mice showed that practicing intermittent fasting for 11 months improved both brain function and brain structure.

Other animal studies have reported that fasting could protect brain health and increase the generation of nerve cells to help enhance cognitive function.

Because fasting may also help relieve inflammation, it could also aid in preventing neurodegenerative disorders.

In particular, studies in animals suggest that fasting may protect against and improve outcomes for conditions such as Alzheimer's disease and Parkinson's. However, more studies are needed to evaluate the effects of fasting on brain function in humans.

Summary Animal studies show that fasting could improve brain function, increase nerve cell synthesis and protect against neurodegenerative conditions, such as Alzheimer's disease and Parkinson's.

5. Aids Weight Loss by Limiting Calorie Intake and Boosting Metabolism

Many dieters pick up fasting looking for a quick and easy way to drop a few pounds.

Theoretically, abstaining from all or certain foods and beverages should decrease your overall calorie intake, which could lead to increased weight loss over time.

Some research has also found that short-term fasting may boost metabolism by increasing levels of the neurotransmitter norepinephrine, which could enhance weight loss.

In fact, one review showed that whole-day fasting could reduce body weight by up to 9% and significantly decrease body fat over 12–24 weeks.

Another review found that intermittent fasting over 3–12 weeks was as effective in inducing weight loss as continuous calorie restriction and decreased body weight and fat mass by up to 8% and 16% respectively.

In addition, fasting was found to be more effective than calorie restriction at increasing fat loss while simultaneously preserving muscle tissue.

Summary

Fasting may increase metabolism and help preserve muscle tissue to reduce body weight and body fat.

6. Increases Growth Hormone Secretion, Which Is Vital for Growth, Metabolism, Weight Loss and Muscle Strength

Human growth hormone (HGH) is a type of protein hormone that is central to many aspects of your health.

In fact, research shows that this key hormone is involved in growth, metabolism, weight loss and muscle strength.

Several studies have found that fasting could naturally increase HGH levels.

One study in 11 healthy adults showed that fasting for 24 hours significantly increased levels of HGH.

Another small study in nine men found that fasting for just two days led to a 5-fold increase in the HGH production rate.

Plus, fasting may help maintain steady blood sugar and insulin levels throughout the day, which may further optimize levels of HGH, as some research has found that sustaining increased levels of insulin may reduce HGH levels.

Summary

Studies show that fasting can increase levels of human growth hormone (HGH), an important protein hormone that plays a role in growth, metabolism, weight loss and muscle strength.

7. Could Delay Aging and Extend Longevity

Several animal studies have found promising results on the potential lifespan-extending effects of fasting.

In one study, rats that fasted every other day experienced a delayed rate of aging and lived 83% longer than rats that didn't fast.

Other animal studies have had similar findings, reporting that fasting could be effective in increasing longevity and survival rates.

However, current research is still limited to animal studies. Further studies are needed to understand how fasting may impact longevity and aging in humans.

Summary

Animal studies have found that fasting could delay aging and increase longevity, but human research is still lacking.

8. May Aid in Cancer Prevention and Increase the Effectiveness of Chemotherapy

Animal and test-tube studies indicate that fasting may benefit the treatment and prevention of cancer.

In fact, one rat study found that alternate-day fasting helped block tumor formation.

Similarly, a test-tube study showed that exposing cancer cells to several cycles of fasting was as effective as chemotherapy in delaying tumor growth and increased the effectiveness of chemotherapy drugs on cancer formation.

Unfortunately, most research is limited to the effects of fasting on cancer formation in animals and cells.

Despite these promising findings, additional studies are needed to look at how fasting may influence cancer development and treatment in humans.

How to Start Fasting

Summary

Some animal and test-tube studies suggest that fasting could block tumor development and increase the effectiveness of chemotherapy.

How to Start Fasting

There are many different types of fasts, making it easy to find a method that fits your lifestyle.

Here are a few of the most common types of fasting:

Water fasting: Involves drinking only water for a set amount of time.

Juice fasting: Entails only drinking vegetable or fruit juice for a certain period.

Intermittent fasting: Intake is partially or completely restricted for a few hours up to a few days at a time and a normal diet is resumed on other

days.

Partial fasting: Certain foods or drinks such as processed foods,

animal products or caffeine are eliminated from the diet for a set period.

Calorie restriction: Calories are restricted for a few days every week.

Within these categories are also more specific types of fasts.

For example, intermittent fasting can be broken down into subcategories, such as alternate-day fasting, which involves eating every other day, or time-restricted feeding, which entails limiting intake to just a few hours each day.

To get started, try experimenting with different types of fasting to find what works best for you.

Summary

There are many different ways to practice fasting, which makes it easy to find a method that fits into just about any lifestyle. Experiment with different types to find what works best for you.

Safety and Side Effects

Despite the long list of possible health benefits associated with fasting, it may not be right for everyone.

If you suffer from diabetes or low blood sugar, fasting can lead to spikes and crashes in your blood sugar levels, which could be dangerous.

It's best to talk to your doctor first if you have any underlying health conditions or are planning to fast for more than 24 hours.

Additionally, fasting is not generally recommended without medical supervision for older adults, adolescents or people who are underweight.

If you decide to try fasting, be sure to stay well-hydrated and fill your diet with nutrient-dense foods during your eating periods to maximize the potential health benefits.

Additionally, if fasting for longer periods, try to minimize intense physical activity and get plenty of rest.

Summary

When fasting, be sure to stay hydrated, eat nutrient-dense foods and get plenty of rest. It's best to consult with your doctor before fasting if you have any underlying health conditions or are planning to fast for more than 24 hours.

The Bottom Line

Fasting is a practice that has been associated with a wide array of potential health benefits, including weight loss, as well as improved blood sugar control, heart health, brain function and cancer prevention.

From water fasting to intermittent fasting and calorie restriction, there are many different types of fasting that fit nearly every lifestyle.

When coupled with a nutritious diet and healthy lifestyle, incorporating fasting into your routine could benefit your health.

Alternate-Day Fasting

Alternate-day fasting is one way to do intermittent fasting.

On this diet, you fast every other day but eat whatever you want on the non-fasting days.

The most common version of this diet involves "modified" fasting, where you can eat around 500 calories on fasting days.

Alternate-day fasting may help promote weight loss and may help lower risk factors related to heart disease and type 2 diabetes.

Here's a detailed beginner's guide to alternate-day fasting.

How to do alternate-day fasting

Alternate-day fasting (ADF) is an intermittent fasting approach.

The basic idea is that you fast on one day and then eat what you want the next day.

This way you only need to restrict what you eat half of the time.

On fasting days, you're allowed to drink as many calorie-free beverages as you like. Examples include:

- water
- unsweetened coffee
- tea

If you're following a modified ADF approach, you're also allowed to eat about 500 calories on fasting days, or 20–25% of your energy requirements.

The most popular version of this diet is called "The Every Other Day Diet" by Dr. Krista Varady, who has conducted most of the studies on ADF.

The health and weight loss benefits seem to be the same regardless of whether the fasting-day calories are consumed at lunch or dinner, or as small meals throughout the day.

Some people may find that alternate day fasting is easier to stick to than other types of diets.

However, a yearlong study found that adherence when following alternate day fasting (where calorie intake was reduced to 25% of energy needs on fasting days) was not superior to everyday calorie restriction.

Most of the studies on alternate-day fasting used the modified version, with 500 calories on fasting days. This is considered much more sustainable than doing full fasts on fasting days, but it's just as effective.

In this book, the terms "alternate-day fasting" or "ADF" generally apply to the modified approach with about 500 calories on fasting days.

SUMMARY

Alternate-day fasting cycles between days of fasting and normal eating. The most popular version allows for about 500 calories on fasting days.

Alternate-day fasting and weight loss

Although ADF may be helpful for promoting weight loss, studies have suggested that this type of calorie restriction is no more effective for weight loss than traditional daily calorie restriction.

Studies among adults with overweight and obesity show that engaging in ADF may help you lose 3–8% of your body weight in 2–12 weeks.

Research suggests that this method is not superior to traditional daily calorie restriction for promoting weight loss.

Studies have shown that ADF and daily calorie restriction are equally effective at reducing harmful belly fat and inflammatory markers in those with obesity.

Although ADF may offer benefits for fat loss, recent research shows that ADF is no more effective than traditional calorie restriction for promoting weight loss or preserving muscle mass.

Furthermore, like other types of calorie restriction, weight loss during ADF may be accelerated when combined with increased physical activity.

For example, combining ADF with endurance exercise may cause twice as much weight loss than ADF alone and six times as much weight loss as endurance exercise alone.

Regarding diet composition, ADF seems to be equally effective whether it's done with a high or low fat diet.

SUMMARY

Alternate-day fasting may help you lose weight. However, research has shown that it's likely no more effective for promoting weight loss than traditional daily calorie restriction.

Alternate-day fasting and hunger

The effects of ADF on hunger are rather inconsistent.

Some studies show that hunger ultimately goes down on fasting days, while others state that hunger remains unchanged.

However, research agrees that modified ADF with 500 calories on fasting days is much more tolerable than full fasts on fasting days.

One study comparing ADF to calorie restriction showed that ADF increased levels of brain-derived neurotrophic factor (BDNF) after 24 weeks of follow- up.

BDNF is a protein that plays a role in energy balance and body weight maintenance.

Researchers concluded that ADF may induce long-term changes in BDNF and that this may promote improved weight loss maintenance.

However, the researchers found that BDNF levels did not correlate with body weight changes in this particular study and suggested that these findings be interpreted with caution.

Human studies have not shown significant effects of ADF on hunger hormones.

However, animal studies have shown that modified ADF resulted in decreased amounts of hunger hormones and increased amounts of satiety hormones compared to other diets.

Another factor to consider is compensatory hunger, which is a frequent downside of traditional, daily calorie restriction.

Compensatory hunger refers to increased levels of hunger in response to calorie restriction, which cause people to eat more than they need to when they finally allow themselves to eat.

Studies have shown that ADF doesn't seem to increase compensatory hunger.

In fact, many people who try modified ADF claim that their hunger diminishes after the first 2 weeks or so. After a while, some find that the fasting days are nearly effortless.

However, the effects of ADF on hunger most likely vary by individual.

SUMMARY

The effects of alternate-day fasting on hunger are inconsistent. Studies on modified alternate-day fasting show that hunger decreases as you adapt to the diet.

Alternate-day fasting and body composition

ADF has been shown to have unique effects on body composition, both while you're dieting and during your weight-maintenance period.

Studies comparing traditional calorie-restricted diets and ADF show that they're equally effective at decreasing weight and fat mass.

Some studies have suggested that ADF may be more beneficial for preserving muscle mass than other types of calorie restriction,

However, results from a recent, high-quality study suggest that ADF is no more effective for preserving muscle mass than traditional calorie restriction.

SUMMARY

Studies suggest that although ADF may help preserve lean muscle mass during weight loss, it's no more effective than other methods of calorie restriction.

Health benefits of alternate-day fasting

ADF has several health benefits aside from weight loss.

Type 2 diabetes

Type 2 diabetes accounts for 90–95% of diabetes cases in the United States.

What's more, more than one-third of Americans have prediabetes, a condition in which blood sugar levels are higher than normal but not high enough to be considered diabetes.

Losing weight and restricting calories is usually an effective way to improve or reverse many symptoms of type 2 diabetes.

Similarly to continuous calorie restriction, ADF seems to cause mild reductions in risk factors for type 2 diabetes among people with overweight or obesity.

ADF may also help reduce fasting insulin levels, with some studies suggesting that it may be more effective than daily calorie restriction.

However, not all studies agree that ADF is superior to daily calorie restriction.

Having high insulin levels, or hyperinsulinemia, has been linked to obesity and chronic diseases, such as heart disease and cancer

A reduction in insulin levels and insulin resistance should lead to a significantly reduced risk of type 2 diabetes, especially when combined with weight loss.

SUMMARY

Alternate-day fasting may reduce risk factors for type 2 diabetes. It can reduce fasting insulin levels in people with prediabetes.

Heart health

Heart disease is the leading cause of death in the world and responsible for about one in four deaths.

Many studies have shown that ADF is a good option to help individuals with overweight or obesity lose weight and reduce heart disease risk factors.

Studies on the subject range from 8–52 weeks and involve those with overweight and obesity.

The most common health benefits include:

- reduced waist circumference (2–2.8 inches or 5–7 cm)
- decreased blood pressure
- lowered LDL (bad) cholesterol (20–25%)
- increased number of large LDL particles and reduced number of dangerous small, dense LDL particles
- decreased blood triglycerides (up to 30%)

SUMMARY

Alternate-day fasting may reduce waist circumference and decrease blood pressure, LDL (bad) cholesterol, and triglycerides.

Alternate-day fasting and autophagy

One of the most common effects of fasting is the stimulation of autophagy.

Autophagy is a process in which old parts of cells are degraded and recycled. It plays a key role in preventing diseases, including cancer, neurodegeneration, heart disease, and infections.

Animal studies have consistently shown that long- and short-term fasting increase autophagy and are linked to delayed aging and a reduced risk of tumors.

Furthermore, fasting has been shown to increase lifespan in rodents, flies, yeasts, and worms.

Moreover, cell studies have shown that fasting stimulates autophagy, resulting in effects that may help keep you healthy and live longer.

This has been supported by human studies showing that ADF diets reduce oxidative damage and promote changes that may be linked to longevity.

The findings look promising, but the effects of ADF on autophagy and longevity need to be studied more extensively.

SUMMARY

Alternate-day fasting stimulates autophagy in animal and cell studies. This process may slow aging and help prevent diseases like cancer and heart disease.

Does alternate-day fasting induce starvation mode?
Nearly all weight loss methods cause a slight drop in resting metabolic rate.

This effect is often referred to as starvation mode, but the technical term is adaptive thermogenesis.

When you severely restrict your calories, your body starts conserving energy by reducing the number of calories it burns. It can make you stop losing weight and feel miserable.

However, ADF doesn't seem to cause this drop in metabolic rate.

One 8-week study compared the effects of standard calorie restriction and ADF.

The results showed that continuous calorie restriction significantly decreased resting metabolic rate by 6% when calculated relative to lean mass, while ADF only caused an insignificant 1% reduction.

What's more, after 24 unsupervised weeks, the calorie restriction group still had a 4.5% lower resting metabolic rate than at the beginning of the study. Meanwhile, the ADF participants experienced only a 1.8% reduction.

SUMMARY

Alternate-day fasting may not decrease metabolic rate in the same way as continuous calorie restriction.

Is it also good for people who are within a normal weight range?

ADF is not only beneficial for weight loss, but it can also offer health benefits for those who don't have obesity.

A 3-week study analyzed individuals with average weight following a strict ADF diet with zero calories on fasting days.

The researchers found that it resulted in increased fat burning, decreased fasting insulin, and a 4% decrease in fat mass.

However, hunger levels remained quite high throughout the study.

They speculated whether a modified ADF diet with one small meal on fasting days might be more tolerable for people who don't have obesity.

Another controlled study involved individuals with overweight and average weight.

It showed that following an ADF diet for 12 weeks reduced fat mass and produced favorable changes in risk factors for heart disease.

That said, ADF generally provides much fewer calories than you need to maintain weight, which is the reason you ultimately lose weight.

If you're not looking to lose weight or fat mass, or have average weight to begin with, other dietary methods will probably suit you better.

SUMMARY

Alternate-day fasting increases fat burning and reduces risk factors for heart disease in people with average weight.

What to eat and drink on fasting days

There's no general rule regarding what you should eat or drink on fasting days, except that your total calorie intake shouldn't exceed around 500 calories.

It's best to drink low calorie or calorie-free drinks on fasting days, such as:

- water
- coffee
- tea

Most people find it best to eat one "big" meal late in the day, while others prefer to eat early or split the amount between 2–3 meals.

Since your calorie intake will be severely limited, it's best to focus on nutritious, high protein foods, as well as low calorie vegetables. These will make you feel full without many calories.

Soups may also be a good option on fasting days, as they tend to make you feel fuller than if you ate the ingredients on their own.

Here are a few examples of meals that are suitable for fasting days:

- eggs and vegetables
- yogurt with berries
- grilled fish or lean meat with vegetables
- soup and a piece of fruit
- a generous salad with lean meat

You can find numerous recipes for quick 500-calorie meals and healthy low calorie snacks online.

SUMMARY

There are no strict guidelines regarding what to eat and drink on fasting days. It's best to stick to high protein foods and vegetables, as well as low calorie or calorie-free beverages.

Is alternate-day fasting safe?

Studies have shown that alternate-day fasting is safe for most people.

It doesn't result in a greater risk for weight regain than traditional, calorie-restricted diets.

Some think that ADF increases your risk of binge eating, but studies have found that it may help reduce binge eating behavior and decrease depressive symptoms.

It may also improve restrictive eating and body image perception among people with obesity. However, more research on the effectiveness and safety of ADF in people with disordered eating tendencies is needed.

That said, ADF is likely not appropriate for certain populations.

These include children, pregnant and lactating women, people who are underweight, and those with certain medical conditions that may be exacerbated by fasting like Gilbert Syndrome.

Although some research suggests that ADF may be helpful for reducing symptoms of binge eating, this dietary pattern is likely not appropriate for people with eating disorders, including anorexia nervosa or bulimia.

Be sure to consult a healthcare provider before trying this eating pattern if you have a medical condition or are currently taking any medications.

SUMMARY

Alternate-day fasting is safe for most people. Consult a healthcare provider to learn if alternate-day fasting is right for you.

The bottom line

Alternate-day fasting is a very effective way to lose weight for most people. It is not recommended for children, people with eating disorders, or those who are pregnant, lactating, or living with rare disorders like Gilbert Syndrome.

It may have benefits over traditional calorie-restricted diets in some cases. It's also linked to major improvements in many health markers.

The best part of all is that it's surprisingly easy to stick to, as you only need to "diet" every other day.

.

Evidence-Based Health Benefits of Intermittent Fasting

Intermittent fasting is an eating pattern where you cycle between periods of eating and fasting.

There are many different types of intermittent fasting, such as the 16/8 or 5:2 methods.

Numerous studies show that it can have powerful benefits for your body and brain.

Here are 10 evidence-based health benefits of intermittent fasting.

1. Intermittent Fasting Changes The Function of Cells, Genes and Hormones

When you don't eat for a while, several things happen in your body.

For example, your body initiates important cellular repair processes and changes hormone levels to make stored body fat more accessible.

Here are some of the changes that occur in your body during fasting:

Insulin levels: Blood levels of insulin drop significantly, which facilitates fat burning.

Human growth hormone: The blood levels of growth hormone may increase as much as 5-fold. Higher levels of this hormone facilitate fat burning and muscle gain, and have numerous other benefits.

Cellular repair: The body induces important cellular repair processes, such as removing waste material from cells.

Gene expression: There are beneficial changes in several genes and molecules related to longevity and protection against disease.

Many of the benefits of intermittent fasting are related to these changes in hormones, gene expression and function of cells.

BOTTOM LINE:

When you fast, insulin levels drop and human growth hormone increases. Your cells also initiate important cellular repair processes and change which genes they express.

2. Intermittent Fasting Can Help You Lose Weight and Belly Fat

Many of those who try intermittent fasting are doing it in order to lose weight.

Generally speaking, intermittent fasting will make you eat fewer meals.

Unless if you compensate by eating much more during the other meals, you will end up taking in fewer calories.

Additionally, intermittent fasting enhances hormone function to facilitate weight loss.

Lower insulin levels, higher growth hormone levels and increased amounts of norepinephrine (noradrenaline) all increase the breakdown of body fat and facilitate its use for energy.

For this reason, short-term fasting actually increases your metabolic rate by 3.6-14%, helping you burn even more calories.

In other words, intermittent fasting works on both sides of the calorie equation. It boosts your metabolic rate (increases calories out) and reduces the amount of food you eat (reduces calories in).

According to a 2014 review of the scientific literature, intermittent fasting can cause weight loss of 3-8% over 3-24 weeks. This is a huge amount.

The people also lost 4-7% of their waist circumference, which indicates that they lost lots of belly fat, the harmful fat in the abdominal cavity that causes disease.

One review study also showed that intermittent fasting caused less muscle loss than continuous calorie restriction.

All things considered, intermittent fasting can be an incredibly powerful weight loss tool.

BOTTOM LINE:

Intermittent fasting helps you eat fewer calories, while boosting metabolism slightly. It is a very effective tool to lose weight and belly fat.

3. Intermittent Fasting Can Reduce Insulin Resistance, Lowering Your Risk of Type 2 Diabetes

Type 2 diabetes has become incredibly common in recent decades.

Its main feature is high blood sugar levels in the context of insulin resistance.

Anything that reduces insulin resistance should help lower blood sugar levels and protect against type 2 diabetes.

Interestingly, intermittent fasting has been shown to have major benefits for insulin resistance and lead to an impressive reduction in blood sugar levels.

In human studies on intermittent fasting, fasting blood sugar has been reduced by 3-6%, while fasting insulin has been reduced by 20-31%.

One study in diabetic rats also showed that intermittent fasting protected against kidney damage, one of the most severe complications of diabetes.

What this implies, is that intermittent fasting may be highly protective for people who are at risk of developing type 2 diabetes.

However, there may be some differences between genders. One study in women showed that blood sugar control actually worsened after a 22-day long intermittent fasting protocol.

BOTTOM LINE:

Intermittent fasting can reduce insulin resistance and lower blood sugar levels, at least in men.

4. Intermittent Fasting Can Reduce Oxidative Stress and Inflammation in The Body

Oxidative stress is one of the steps towards aging and many chronic diseases.

It involves unstable molecules called free radicals, which react with other important molecules (like protein and DNA) and damage them.

Several studies show that intermittent fasting may enhance the body's resistance to oxidative stress.

Additionally, studies show that intermittent fasting can help fight inflammation, another key driver of all sorts of common diseases.

BOTTOM LINE:

Studies show that intermittent fasting can reduce oxidative damage and inflammation in the body. This should have benefits against aging and development of numerous diseases.

5. Intermittent Fasting May be Beneficial For Heart Health

Heart disease is currently the world's biggest killer.

It is known that various health markers (so-called "risk factors") are associated with either an increased or decreased risk of heart disease.

Intermittent fasting has been shown to improve numerous different risk factors, including blood pressure, total and LDL cholesterol, blood triglycerides, inflammatory markers and blood sugar levels.

However, a lot of this is based on animal studies. The effects on heart health need to be studied a lot further in humans before recommendations can be made.

BOTTOM LINE:

Studies show that intermittent fasting can improve numerous risk factors for heart disease such as blood pressure, cholesterol levels, triglycerides and inflammatory markers.

6. Intermittent Fasting Induces Various Cellular Repair Processes

When we fast, the cells in the body initiate a cellular "waste removal" process called autophagy.

This involves the cells breaking down and metabolizing broken and dysfunctional proteins that build up inside cells over time.

Increased autophagy may provide protection against several diseases, including cancer and Alzheimer's disease.

BOTTOM LINE:

Fasting triggers a metabolic pathway called autophagy, which removes waste material from cells.

7. Intermittent Fasting May Help Prevent Cancer

Cancer is a terrible disease, characterized by uncontrolled growth of cells.

Fasting has been shown to have several beneficial effects on metabolism that may lead to reduced risk of cancer.

Although human studies are needed, promising evidence from animal studies indicates that intermittent fasting may help prevent cancer.

There is also some evidence on human cancer patients, showing that fasting reduced various side effects of chemotherapy.

BOTTOM LINE:

Intermittent fasting has been shown to help prevent cancer in animal studies. One paper in humans showed that it can reduce side effects caused by chemotherapy.

8. Intermittent Fasting is Good For Your Brain

What is good for the body is often good for the brain as well.

Intermittent fasting improves various metabolic features known to be important for brain health.

This includes reduced oxidative stress, reduced inflammation and a reduction in blood sugar levels and insulin resistance.

Several studies in rats have shown that intermittent fasting may increase the growth of new nerve cells, which should have benefits for brain function. It also increases levels of a brain hormone called brain-derived neurotrophic factor (BDNF), a deficiency of which has been implicated in depression and various other brain problems.

Animal studies have also shown that intermittent fasting protects against brain damage due to strokes.

BOTTOM LINE:

Intermittent fasting may have important benefits for brain health. It may increase growth of new neurons and protect the brain from damage.

9. Intermittent Fasting May Help Prevent Alzheimer's Disease

Alzheimer's disease is the world's most common neurodegenerative disease.

There is no cure available for Alzheimer's, so preventing it from showing up in the first place is critical.

A study in rats shows that intermittent fasting may delay the onset of Alzheimer's disease or reduce its severity.

In a series of case reports, a lifestyle intervention that included daily short-term fasts was able to significantly improve Alzheimer's symptoms in 9 out of 10 patients.

Animal studies also suggest that fasting may protect against other neurodegenerative diseases, including Parkinson's and Huntington's disease.

However, more research in humans is needed.

BOTTOM LINE:

Studies in animals suggest that intermittent fasting may be protective against neurodegenerative diseases like Alzheimer's disease.

10. Intermittent Fasting May Extend Your Lifespan, Helping You Live Longer

One of the most exciting applications of intermittent fasting may be its ability to extend lifespan.

Studies in rats have shown that intermittent fasting extends lifespan in a similar way as continuous calorie restriction.

In some of these studies, the effects were quite dramatic. In one of them, rats that fasted every other day lived 83% longer than rats who weren't fasted.

Although this is far from being proven in humans, intermittent fasting has become very popular among the anti-aging crowd.

Given the known benefits for metabolism and all sorts of health markers, it makes sense that intermittent fasting could help you live a longer and healthier life.